I0396822

Essential Oils and Aromatherapy

Beginners Guide to Natural Healing, Weight Loss, and Stress Relief

Copyright 2015 by: Cassandra Slain, All rights reserved.

This document is geared towards providing exact and reliable information in regards to the topic and issue covered. The publication is sold with the idea that the publisher is not required to render accounting, officially permitted, or otherwise, qualified services. If advice is necessary, legal or professional, a practiced individual in the profession should be ordered.

From a Declaration of Principles which was accepted and approved equally by a Committee of the American Bar Association and a Committee of Publishers and Associations.

In no way is it legal to reproduce, duplicate, or transmit any part of this document in either electronic means or in printed format. Recording of this publication is strictly prohibited and any storage of this document is not allowed unless with written permission from the publisher. All rights reserved.

The information provided herein is stated to be truthful and consistent, in that any liability, in terms of inattention or otherwise, by any usage or abuse of any policies, processes, or directions contained within is the solitary and utter responsibility of the recipient reader. Under no circumstances will any legal responsibility or blame be held against the publisher for any reparation, damages, or monetary loss due to the information herein, either directly or indirectly.

Respective authors own all copyrights not held by the publisher.

The information herein is offered for informational purposes solely, and is universal as so. The presentation of the information is without contract or any type of guarantee assurance.

The trademarks that are used are without any consent, and the publication of the trademark is without permission or backing by the trademark owner. All trademarks and brands within this book are for clarifying purposes only and are the owned by the owners themselves, not affiliated with this document.

Thanks for reading!

Introduction

Over the past few decades, there has been a growing interest in folk remedies and alternative treatments. This has led many people to seek out these alternatives to conventional medicine. These alternative treatments range from herbal remedies to acupressure - and even psychic healing.

These kinds of treatments are, for the most part, not new, and have always existed in some form or another. While a few, like Homeopathy, are fairly recent developments, folk remedies using herbs have been around for millennia. Acupressure has been practiced in countries such as China for ages. Psychic healing has also been a part of many cultures around the world for a very long time.

People have a variety of perspectives on alternative treatments. Some believe these treatments have worked for them. Other people have seen no benefits from herbal folk remedies.

Even the scientific and medical communities are divided on their approach to these forms of alternative medicine. Experts in these fields have attitudes toward aromatherapy that range from indecision to complete opposition. However, few studies have been undertaken done to test the claims of these various treatments.

Despite this, many people around the world continue to use traditional remedies. Some rely solely on alternative treatments while others use them alongside conventional medicines. Until more tests are done, people are mostly left on their own to decide whether or not to use a particular form of alternative medicine.

This book will introduce you to one form of alternative treatment, aromatherapy. It discusses the practices and beliefs of aromatherapy, how this technique uses essential oils and other plant materials, and why aromatherapy practitioners believe it can be used for healing, weight loss, and stress relief. This book also provides suggestions for the use of essential oils in your home.

However, just like everyone else who has studied alternative forms of treatment - once you have been completely informed, the choice to use these methods (or not) is yours to make. So, use your mind and your intuition, and welcome to the study of aromatherapy!

Table of Contents

Chapter One: What Is Aromatherapy?

Ask a number of different people about aromatherapy, and you'll probably receive many different answers. The less informed may say that it's a way to use fragrances to heal sickness. Those who practice a more holistic form of aromatherapy may claim that it's a natural form of medicine that uses essential oils to bring about complete wholeness and health. Other practitioners of aromatherapy may provide answers that lie somewhere between these two extremes.

Aromatherapy is the practice of using aromatic plant materials such as essential oils to treat physical or psychological disorders, improve mood, or increase cognitive function. Aside from essential oils, aromatherapists also make use of absolutes, carrier oils, distillates, and infusions during treatment.

Aromatherapy generally makes use of plant oils, and can be considered an offshoot of herbal medicine. In fact, more than a few of the properties assigned to certain essential oils come from various herbal medicine practices around the world.

Despite its name, aromatherapy isn't only concerned with the scent or fragrance of the oils used. The oil itself plays an important part in treatment.

Aromatherapy is believed to work in two ways. The first is through the inhalation of the fragrance. This effect is carried through a person's olfactory system to the rest of the body. The second method of transmission is by absorption through the skin. This is accomplished by direct application, baths, or massage.

A professional aromatherapist chooses an application method depending on the type of oil, the purpose of the treatment, and their personal experience, beliefs, and practices.

Scents in the Ancient World

While the term "aromatherapy" has been in use for less than a century, plant materials such as essential oils have been used for their fragrance and medicinal properties since ancient times. For millennia, fragrances have been used in religious rituals, including healing ceremonies.

In Ancient Egypt, a variety of aromatic plant materials were used to treat a wide range of conditions, from skin diseases to respiratory problems. Various fragrances were also used in Ancient Egyptian religious rituals - and in the embalming process.

In Ancient India, essential oils were combined with massage and a form of acupressure, which was said to promote health and healing. This traditional medicine still exists in some forms today. These practices have been incorporated into a number of alternative medical treatments, of which aromatherapy is only one of many.

Aromatic medicine was part of the ancient medical practices that evolved into what we know as Chinese acupuncture. These practices are still in use today; China's traditional herbal medicine and acupuncture are some of the most accepted forms of alternative medicine.

In Ancient Greece, Hippocrates, the father of medicine, studied hundreds of plants for their medicinal properties and advocated daily aromatic baths. Ancient Rome was heavily influenced by the practices and knowledge of the Egyptians and Greeks. The Romans made use of therapeutic massages with aromatic oils to treat a range of conditions, including the common cold.

In Arabia, various herbal medicines were widely used. These included various aromatic medicines distilled from plants. This knowledge traveled and spread throughout Europe during the time of the Crusades. In the Middle Ages, lavender, frankincense, and pine were burned in the streets of European cities to combat the Bubonic plague and mask the scent of the dead.

Modern Aromatherapy

The term "aromatherapy" was first used in 1937 by French chemist Rene-Maurice Gattefosse. In his book, *Aromatherapy*, he explains how he used lavender essential oil to treat a severe burn he sustained while working in his laboratory. This led him to experiment on the healing properties of essential oils.

Another Frenchman, Dr. Jean Valnet, continued the research done by Gattefosse. During World War II, he used essential oils as antiseptics to treat wounded soldiers. In 1964, he published the book *Practice of Aromatherapy*, a work that is considered by many aromatherapists to be the "Bible" of aromatherapy.

Today, aromatherapy is used to treat sickness, improve physical and mental health, relax the mind, and ease stress. Some practitioners use it alongside conventional medical treatments while others use it as an alternative to treatment. Others simply use essential oils to relax after a long day.

The Tools of Aromatherapy

Most people know that aromatherapists use essential oils but are less aware of the other plant materials and oils used in aromatherapy.

Absolutes are similar to essential oils; they are both concentrated, fragrant oils extracted from plants. The main difference between absolutes and essential oils is that absolutes are produced through solvent extraction, or "enfleurage".

Carrier oils or "base oils" are plant oils combined with essential oils and absolutes. This process dilutes these potent oils before application to the skin. Carrier oils are essential to preparing essential oils for massage therapy. Carrier oils generally do not have a strong fragrance.

Herbal distillates are the liquid byproducts of the distillation process used to extract essential oils. They contain essential oils and other plant acids and are typically less irritating to the skin than pure essential oils.

Infusions are created by suspending plant materials in solvents, such as water, alcohol, or oil. The time spent in the solvent often depends on what the infusion will be used for.

Chapter Two: Essential Oils

Essential oils are plant oils, typically extracted by means of distillation from different parts of aromatic plants. These oils are called "essential" because they contain the essential fragrances and properties of the plants they were extracted from. Aside from aromatherapy, essential oils are also used to provide fragrance to perfumes, soaps, and cleaning products. They have also been used to add flavor to food and drink.

Typically non-soluble in water, essential oils are usually diluted in oil, fat, or pure alcohol before being used to add fragrance to products. In the practice of aromatherapy, however, vegetable oils called "carrier oils" are used for this purpose.

Scientists identify many chemicals that give essential oils their aromas, making it possible to create synthetic fragrant oils. These synthetic oils smell much the same as the essential oils they were based on. However, many aromatherapists believe these synthetic fragrances do not have the same potency as essential oils.

The purity of essential oils is very important to aromatherapists, and some will refuse to work with anything other than 100% pure, natural essential oils. Other aromatherapists are less strict, making use of oils, candles, and incense made from synthetic fragrances.

Extraction of Essential Oils

Essential oils are usually only extracted one parts a plant, such as the flowers, leaves, or fruit. In some cases, however, essential oils may be extracted from different parts of the same plant.

The amount of plant material required to create a certain amount of essential oil varies from plant to plant. This factor affects the cost and rarity of the essential oil. In some cases, as much as one hundred kilos of plant material are required to produce just one liter of essential oil.

Distillation

The primary method of extracting essential oils is through distillation. In this process, plant material is placed in a still and heated by water or steam. This causes the cells of the plant to break open and free the essential oils. The essential oils and steam are then channeled into a cooling tank where the water and oil are separated. After the removal of the essential oil, a fragrant byproduct called an "herbal distillate" remains, which is sometimes used in aromatherapy.

Distillation requires great skill and knowledge of the specific plants involved. Some plants need to be distilled immediately after harvesting while others need to be dried first. Different plants also require different distillation temperatures and times.

Expression

Before the discovery of distillation, expression was the only method available for extracting essential oils. Though it is done today by mechanical presses, expression was historically done by hand. The liquid collected by pressing is filtered to get pure essential oil. Today, this method is mainly used on citrus peels because they contain high amounts of essential oils and do not need to be distilled.

Solvent Extraction

When a plant's oils are too delicate to survive the high heat used in distillation, the process of solvent extraction is used instead. Solvent extraction involves covering the aromatic plant material with a solvent, creating a blend of wax and oil called a "concrete". This concrete is mixed with alcohol, chilled, and filtered. The alcohol is allowed to evaporate slowly, leaving behind only the plant oils, called an "absolute".

Absolutes are very similar to essential oils and are used in much the same way. However, the process of solvent extraction can leave trace amounts of impurities in the absolute. Because of this, some aromatherapists avoid their use.

Care and Storage

Essential oils need to be handled with great care and stored properly. They are sensitive to air, light, temperature, and age, and these four factors should always be kept in mind when handling essential oils.

Air: Essential oils are volatile and tend to evaporate - even at normal temperatures. Lighter, more viscous oils tend to evaporate faster. However, even denser essential oils will evaporate over time if their container is not air-tight. Exposure to air can change the aroma of essential oils and diminish their therapeutic value.

Light: Many essential oils can be damaged by ultraviolet light, which is why most are sold in dark or amber-colored glass bottles. Even then, it is best to store them in a dark place, and never place them in direct sunlight.

Temperature: Extremes of temperature can affect essential oils and can make them more viscous and cloudy. It is best to store them where the temperature is neither too hot nor too cold. In addition to this, essential oils are highly flammable, and should never be used around open flames.

Age: Even if they are stored in a dark place at the proper temperature, essential oils still lose their efficacy with age. They have varying shelf lives (often from two to three years), after which they should no longer be used. Some aromatherapists claim that certain essential oils get better with age, but there is little agreement in regard to this. Blended or diluted essential oils have an even shorter shelf-life, and should be used within six months after dilution.

Chapter Three: Methods of Treatment

Aromatherapy uses fragrances and essential oils in a number of ways. Treatment will often involve one or more of the following methods, and make use of at least one kind of essential oil. The exact method and fragrances used will depend on the treatment required and the diagnosis of the aromatherapist.

Inhalation

Inhalation is believed to be the quickest way for essential oils to affect the body. This method is commonly used for respiratory problems. Inhalation is also useful when essential oils are used to affect a person's mood.

There are a variety of inhalation methods:

Direct Inhalation: Some aromatherapists recommend inhaling directly from a bottle of essential oils. Others tell patients to place a few drops on a handkerchief (or tissue) and inhale through this cloth to get immediate relief from coughs and colds.

Steam Inhalation: This variation makes use of a few drops of essential oil in a bowl of warm, hot, or boiling water. The patient leans over the bowl for up to fifteen minutes. A towel can be placed over the patient's head to help direct the steam. The patient should keep their eyes closed while leaning over the bowl to avoid possible irritation.

Aerial Diffusion: This method of inhalation can be used to disinfect a room and make it more fragrant. It is often used when a room will be used for a long period of time, such as for sleeping, resting or working. Depending on the essential oil used, this can make a room either more calming or more energizing. A few drops of essential oil mixed with water are enough to diffuse a fragrance through a room for hours. However, some practitioners also use incense for aerial diffusion.

Direct Application

This is most often used for skin care or relaxation, but can also help to treat skin irritations and injuries such as cuts and bruises. These methods are quite popular, and can usually be found in spas that offer aromatherapy treatments.

Aromatic Bath: This method can be used to treat skin irritations or promote relaxation. If using a bathtub, it should be filled with warm water before adding a few drops of essential oil. The patient should then soak for ten to fifteen minutes, allowing the essential oils to be absorbed through the skin.

Hand or Foot Bath: This is an alternative to an aromatic bath if a bathtub is unavailable or impractical to use, or if the hands and feet are the target area. A warm bowl is filled with enough warm water to completely submerge the hands or feet. A few drops of essential oil are added, and the patient soaks the targeted limbs for ten to fifteen minutes.

Compress: Hot or cold compresses can be used to treat muscle aches, arthritis pain, headaches, and similar ailments. They can also be used to treat fevers. Hot compresses should be used for chronic pain. Cold compresses are best for treating painful, inflamed areas. A small bowl is filled with water of the proper temperature, and a few drops of essential oil are added in. A small towel can then be soaked in the solution and applied to the painful areas.

Massage: While essential oils should never be applied directly to the skin, they can be used in massage when mixed with a carrier oil. Aromatherapists often have a preferred carrier oil for massages (usually a kind of vegetable oil), which they mix with precise amounts of essential oils. Massages can be used to influence mood, relieve stress, and alleviate muscle and joint pain. They can be used over the entire body, or targeted at specific areas in need of relief.

Ingestion

Essential oils are not typically ingested; a number of them are very toxic when taken internally. Few aromatherapists will recommend ingestion as a means of treatment, and most will advise against it. Even when an aromatherapist does recommend it, great care is taken when creating the dilution to be used. Never ingest an essential oil without consulting your doctor and a professional aromatherapist.

Mouthwash: Though gargling is not complete ingestion, essential oils are still taken internally through this method (though most of the oil/water mixture is spat out afterward). These mouthwashes are created by adding a drop or two of an essential oil to half a glass of water. The patient then gargles this mixture one mouthful at a time. Just like with full ingestion, get expert advice before attempting to gargle with essential oil mixtures.

Chapter Four: Alternative Vs. Complementary

There is much debate about the use and efficacy of aromatherapy. Though modern aromatherapy was originated and developed by chemists, aromatherapy also includes many practices from herbal alternative medicine. Because many claims about the properties of essential oils aren't grounded in scientific fact, this leads many people to question whether or not they really work.

You might think there's a simple answer to this question. However, the answer is much more complex than "yes" or "no".

Alternative Therapy

Many aromatherapists advocate the use of aromatherapy as a complete and effective alternative to conventional medicine. Most of them point to the long history of the use of herbal remedies in countries such as China, as well as the many testimonials of those who have used aromatherapy to successfully treat their illnesses. Often, these aromatherapists believe in the power of holistic aromatherapy healing. They advocate for treating the whole person—mind, body, and spirit—to get the best health results possible.

Aromatherapists who believe in this use of aromatherapy often believe their approach is superior to conventional medicine. One argument is that conventional medicines always have side effects, while essential oils do not. This belief can lead their patients to believe that they must choose one or the other - either aromatherapy or conventional medicine.

The difficulty with this approach is that there are too few scientific studies to prove the efficacy of the wide range of plant materials and essential oils that aromatherapists use. Also, the spiritual aspects of aromatherapy are unquantifiable by science. Often, patients who choose this form of treatment must take a leap of faith and trust in those who have gone before them - as well as their aromatherapists.

Some will argue that this is no different from the faith and trust patients put in doctors. However, the main difference is that doctors can point to scientific studies to defend their choices of treatment options.

Complementary Therapy

A growing number of aromatherapists, however, take a different approach to aromatherapy - applying it alongside conventional medicine. Often, an aromatherapist works with a medical doctor in order to create a program of care for a patient that involves the use of both conventional medicine and aromatherapy.

Aromatherapy treatments used in concert with conventional medicine are typically aimed at improving mood, alleviating pain, and promoting relaxation. These practitioners use essential oils that have been proven to work alongside conventional treatments. Some may look at this as limiting the possibilities of aromatherapy while others believe it is a more conscientious approach.

As alternative approaches to the treatment of illnesses are further examined by science, more and more alternatives become available to aromatherapists. Already, some scientific studies have pointed to the successful use of aromatherapy in the treatment of hair loss, constipation, itching, and psoriasis. While this does not begin to address all of the many alternative practices of aromatherapy, these are valid diseases for which many patients are grateful to have treatment.

Remember, this debate doesn't have only two sides. Some medical doctors believe aromatherapy is a useful treatment for certain conditions. Likewise, certain holistic practitioners believe aromatherapy is best used as a complementary therapy to conventional medicine. Research into aromatherapy and other alternative treatments continues, and the debate shows no signs of stopping.

The Placebo Effect

Many people believe that aromatherapy and other alternative treatments work only because of the "placebo effect". This refers to treatments or medicine that can work (or appear to work) because the patient believes that they will.

Placebos are often used in medical research. A placebo is given to a control group while the medicine or treatment method being tested is given to an experimental group. The control group should show little to no reaction, and provides a baseline to see if the treatment being tested is effective - and by how much.

The term "placebo effect" has a negative connotation today, especially when referring to alternative treatments. However, the results of many medical studies have shown that even those in a control group can see positive results. Even though these patients are only given a placebo, they sometimes show the effects of treatment.

This has lead to more research on the placebo effect itself, and how it can help the body heal itself. Initial findings are promising. They that the placebo effect can be used to treat various psychological disorders, relieve pain, and perhaps even treat certain heart conditions. Studies are ongoing, and many doctors are considering the ethics of using placebos in their treatment of patients.

The medical community's interest in the placebo effect implies a number of things for alternative treatments like aromatherapy. Firstly, more doctors are willing to consider the use of aromatherapy as a complementary or even an alternative form of treatment. Secondly, even if it's shown that many essential oils are only effective because of the placebo effect, the fact remains that the placebo effect <u>works</u> - and can help the body heal itself. Because many people believe in the efficacy of aromatherapy—placebo or not—they may find healing through its use.

Chapter Five: Commonly Used Essential Oils

Aromatherapy makes use of a wide range of essential oils. The properties of these oils have been studied by alternative herbal medicine practitioners (and, in some cases, scientific researchers). In this chapter, you will discover some of the most commonly used essential oils and learn how they can be used safely. You will find out what precautions you need to take to ensure the safe use of these essential oils.

This list of essential oils is by no means complete, but it should help you begin to choose essential oils for use in your home. However, proper care should always be taken when using them. Unless an oil is considered safe, avoid skin contact with pure oils and completely avoid ingestion (unless directed to do so by a doctor or professional aromatherapist). If skin or eye irritation occurs because of contact with essential oils, wash the area thoroughly with clean water and get in touch with a doctor immediately.

Bergamot: This essential oil is extracted from *Citrus bergamia*, otherwise known as Bergamot orange. The scent of the oil is warm, spicy, and floral and is somewhat similar to lavender. Bergamot oil ranges from green to greenish-yellow in appearance and has a watery consistency.

Bergamot can be used to treat depression and anorexia. It can also relieve stress, tension, and fear. Some people use it for skin infections such as acne and eczema.

This essential oil is photosensitive. Be careful not to expose your skin after treatment - Bergamot oil can dramatically increase your chances of sunburn.

Cedarwood: There are two kinds of cedarwood essential oil: atlas cedarwood and Virginian cedarwood. Atlas cedarwood oil comes from *Cedrus atlantica* while Virginian cedarwood oil comes from *Juniperus virginiana*. These are two completely different species of tree.

Atlas cedarwood smells woody and sweet, with a slight hint of camphor, and has a light golden-yellow color. It can be used to treat acne, dermatitis, and dandruff. It can also help ease coughing and stress.

Virginian cedarwood also has a woody smell, similar to sandalwood, and may be clear to pale-yellow in color. Like atlas cedarwood, it can also be used to treat acne, dermatitis, and dandruff, and may help treat coughing. It may also help in the treatment of arthritis, and can work as an insect repellant.

Atlas Cedarwood is generally safer than Virginian Cedarwood, which may irritate the skin if used in high concentrations. Some sources also claim that oils made from Virginian Cedarwood have carcinogenic properties. Both types of essential oil should be avoided during pregnancy.

Chamomile: There are two kinds of chamomile essential oil: Roman (or "English") Chamomile, which is extracted from *Anthemis nobilis*, and German (or "Hungarian") Chamomile, which is extracted from *Matricaria chamomilla*.

Roman Chamomile essential oil has a fruity, apple-like fragrance and is gray to clear blue in color. German Chamomile essential oil has a sweet, herbal or straw-like scent. German Chamomile has a dark blue color.

Both kinds of chamomile essential oil can be used to treat acne, eczema, dermatitis, and skin allergies. They can also help to soothe irritable children! These oils also relieve abdominal pain (especially in women suffering from PMS), as well as headaches. Chamomile essential oils can be used for throat infections, and are also useful for treating allergies and asthma. Both types are considered non-toxic and non-irritant, but should be avoided during pregnancy.

Eucalyptus: Extracted from Tasmanian blue gum, or *Eucalyptus globulus,* this essential oil has a clear, sharp, eucalyptus smell and a pale yellow color.

This essential oil can help to cool and deodorize the body and can help with fevers and migraines. It can also be used with coughs, throat infections, and other respiratory problems, such as colds and hay fever. It can also be used for muscle pains and rheumatoid arthritis, and can also be used to relieve burns, wounds, skin infections, and insect bites. Eucalyptus oil has also been found to boost the immune system.

Eucalyptus essential oil can cause headaches after excessive use, and should be avoided by those with high blood pressure or epilepsy.

Jasmine: Extracted from various species of jasmine, this oil is actually an "absolute". It has a sweet, floral fragrance. Jasmine typically has a deep brown color, and may have a slight golden tinge.

Jasmine absolutes can help soothe nerves, restore energy, and treat depression. They have also been used to help women during childbirth by strengthening contractions and relieving pain. Jasmine can also be used to treat dry, irritated, and sensitive skin. It is used to reduce scarring and stretch marks, and may restore skin elasticity.

Jasmine oil is generally safe. It is considered non-toxic, non-irritant, and non-sensitizing. However, some people have allergic reactions to this oil.

Lavender: Oils are extracted from many different species of lavender. *Lavandula angustifolia* or *Lavandula officinalis* are most commonly used. The fragrance of lavender oil is light and fresh; this oil has a clear or slightly yellowish color.

Lavender oil is used to relieve stress and calm nerves. It is helpful in treating depression, panic, and hysteria. Lavender is also useful for treating headaches, migraines, and insomnia, and can relieve pain caused by sore muscles, rheumatism, and arthritis. In addition to this, lavender essential oil can help treat asthma, colds, and throat infections, and can also help to ease a person's digestive system.

Lavender can tone and revitalize skin. It also helps with acne, oily skin, sunburn, and wounds. It also acts as an insect repellant and provides relief from insect bites. Lavender oil can be used directly on the skin, and may be used to treat minor burns.

Lemon: Extracted from lemon rinds from the *Citrus limon* plant, this essential oil has the sharp scent of lemon rinds. It can range from pale yellow to deep yellow though it may also be greenish-yellow in appearance.

Lemon essential oil can increase circulation, reduce blood pressure, and boost the immune system. It can also be used to fight fevers and relieve throat infections. Lemon essential oil is soothing, and can relieve headaches and promote relaxation. It may also be applied to the skin to clear acne and other skin irritations - such as insect bites.

Lemon essential oil is non-toxic but can cause allergic reactions in some individuals. It is also photosensitive, and should not be used on the skin before exposure to the sun.

Marjoram: Extracted from knotted marjoram, or *Origanum marjorana,* this essential oil has a warm, spicy smell and is typically colorless. However, it sometimes has a pale yellow to amber color.

Marjoram can be helpful in relieving stress, and has been used to calm even very hyperactive people. It is a muscle relaxant, and can provide relief from rheumatic pain, sore muscles, sprains, and swollen joints. It can be used to soothe cramps, indigestion, constipation, and flatulence, and can also be used to treat colds, sinusitis, and asthma. Marjoram has also been successfully used as a general relaxant to relieve headaches and migraines, and may even help those with insomnia. However, it is also known to diminish sexual desire.

Marjoram essential oil is considered safe, but should not be used during pregnancy.

Peppermint: This oil is extracted from *Mentha piperita*, also known as "brandy mint", or "balm mint". Peppermint oil has a sharp menthol smell (like concentrated peppermint candies) and is usually clear to pale yellow in color.

This essential oil is excellent for treating depression and mental fatigue. It can refresh the spirit and improve concentration. It can also help with shock, headache, migraines, stress, and vertigo. Peppermint oil is used to treat dry coughs, congestion, asthma, and other respiratory disorders, as well as colic, cramps and flatulence. It is even used to relieve pain.

Peppermint oil can relieve skin irritations, itchiness, and other skin conditions while also soothing inflammations. It also cools the skin and can be used to relieve sunburns.

Peppermint oil can applied to the skin in low dilutions, but some people may be sensitive to it. It can cause skin irritations, and should be kept away from the eyes. Peppermint should not be used during pregnancy, or by children under seven.

Rose: Extracted from the Damask Rose (or "Turkish Rose"), *Rosa Damascena*, this oil has a strong floral scent, and may be found either as an essential oil or as an absolute. Rose essential oils are clear to pale yellow in color; rose absolutes are a deep red.

Rose oil is helpful in soothing the mind, and can be helpful in treating depression or grief. It can also relieve stress and other emotional problems. It can improve heart problems, poor circulation, and lower your blood pressure.

Rose oil can help moisturize and hydrate skin, and can also be used as an antiseptic. It is non-toxic, non-irritant, and non-sensitizing, but should be avoided during pregnancy.

Rosemary: There are many species of rosemary, but this essential oil is extracted from *Rosmarinus officinalis*. This essential oil is clear and has a strong, refreshing fragrance that may seem slightly medicinal.

Rosemary oil is said to help improve mental awareness and memory, and can relieve headaches and migraines. It can be used as an antiseptic, but is more often used to treat aching muscles, arthritis, and rheumatism. It is also known to stimulate hair growth and help with other scalp disorders.

People with high blood pressure or epilepsy should avoid rosemary oil, as should those who are pregnant.

Sandalwood: This oil is extracted from East Indian sandalwood, *Santalum album.* Sandalwood oil is pale yellow to gold and has a lingering, delicate, woody scent.

Sandalwood is ideal for treating depression and has a calming effect on many people. It can also treat bronchitis and dry coughs, and may be applied to the skin to relieve itching and inflammation. It is considered a completely safe essential oil, and has been used as a component in many anti-aging skin products.

Tea Tree: This essential oil comes from *Melaleuca alternifolia,* more commonly known as the "narrow-leaved tea tree". This is one of the most commonly used essential oils. It has a light, somewhat medicinal, and spicy scent. The oil itself is often clear with a slight yellow tinge.

Tea tree essential oil is well known as an immuno-stimulant and helps to prevent infection. It has known antibacterial and antifungal properties, and may be used to treat acne, burns, athlete's foot, sunburn, and other skin infections. However, it should not be used internally, or on deep wounds. Avoid contact with the eyes, ears, nose, or mouth.

Ylang-ylang: This essential oil is extracted from ylang-ylang tree, *Cananga odorata,* and has a strong, sweet, floral smell. This oil looks clear with a yellow tinge.

Ylang-ylang has a sedative effect and helps with anxiety, depression, hypertension, and stress. It is also said to have aphrodisiac qualities. When applied to the skin, this oil can regulate the secretion of sebum, making it useful in treating both dry and oily skin. It can also promote hair growth.

The oil is considered safe though excessive use can lead to sensitivity, headaches, and nausea.

Chapter 6: Examples of Use

Aromatherapy may be practiced differently, depending on the aromatherapist. As previously discussed, some practitioners believe in using aromatherapy by itself as a treatment while others work with doctors to provide complementary treatments. Because of these differences in beliefs (and others), aromatherapists have many different approaches to treatment.

Holistic Aromatherapy

The holistic approach to aromatherapy believes that each person is composed of body, mind, and spirit and that these three parts are linked. Something that affects your mind can affect your body, and something that affects your body can affect your mind. With this in mind, the practice of holistic aromatherapy uses essential oils and fragrances to affect, body, mind and spirit in order to treat the whole person, and not just a specific illness.

Aromatherapists who practice a holistic form of aromatherapy will often have lengthy discussions with their patients about not only their conditions, but also about their daily experiences and lifestyles. Only then will the aromatherapist feel confident enough to recommend a treatment program that can treat the whole patient.

Complementary Aromatherapy

Aromatherapists who practice complementary aromatherapy often work with medical doctors to create treatment plans that include both conventional medical treatments and aromatics to improve mood and relieve pain. These aromatherapists will consider the patient's condition and current treatment plan, and will also usually ask the patient what scents and fragrances they prefer. This personal and medical information can affect the kind of essential oils to be used, as well as how they will be applied.

Using Essential Oils At Home

It's possible to practice aromatherapy at home. Aromatherapists recommend some form of home treatment for many conditions. A large number of essential oils are readily available though care should be taken to ensure that the fragrances you purchase are of good quality.

The list in the previous chapter can help you get started, and you can find information online about other essential oils. You will probably want to begin by purchasing and knowing how to use essential oils for minor injuries and burns. After that, you may want to explore oils for relief from headaches, relaxation, and insect bites. However, it's your journey - the oils you familiarize yourself with are yours to choose.

Aside from selecting the oils you want to use, you should also consider where and how you'll be storing them. In addition to this, you may also want to use a clay vaporizer (or a similar device) that diffuses essential oils through the air.

Weight Loss

Most aromatherapists agree that no essential oil can make you instantly lose weight. That being said, a number of essential oils can help you lose weight over time, especially when combined with exercise and a proper diet.

It is said that grapefruit essential oil can help your body dissolve body fat, improve digestion, and stimulate your metabolism. It may be massaged into the skin or taken internally with water. However, be sure to consult an aromatherapist or doctor before doing so.

The fragrances of peppermint and lemon have been found to help manage food cravings, and can be of great help to people on diets.

If you have an exercise plan, you can use essential oils like eucalyptus and lavender to help you feel more energized. On the other hand, chamomile and sandalwood can help you relax as you cool down after exercise.

Essential oils can be very useful in helping you stick to your weight loss plan. Through a combination of diet, exercise, and the use of oils, it is possible to lose weight through aromatherapy.

Stress Relief

This is one of the most common uses of aromatherapy, and one that many people consider totally legitimate. However, a wide range of essential oils can be helpful for relaxation. It is sometimes a matter of personal preference - you'll have to find out for yourself which oil works best for you.

You may apply essential for stress through a clay vaporizer or diffuser, or combine them with a carrier oil for use in a massage. This combination of a calming fragrance and a soothing massage is pretty much guaranteed to help you relieve stress.

Conclusion

All around the world, scents and fragrances play a large part in people's lives. Though we often aren't aware of it, our sense of smell affects our minds, emotions, and bodies in powerful ways. Some scents make us feel safe and secure, like the familiar scents of friends and family members. Some scents help us remember good times, like freshly mowed grass or the hint of a familiar perfume. Other scents can make us recoil, like the smell of spoiled food.

We experience many things in life through scent, like good food and drink, the smell of a new car, or the scent of a newborn baby. It may be hard to explain or quantify, but these effects are powerful and real. Scents can unlock emotions, help us make choices, and change our quality of life.

We can shape our lives and lifestyles through the use of essential oils in aromatherapy. One fragrance can make us feel happy while another can make us feel strong and relaxed. We can even use these essential oils to help our bodies and minds grow healthier.

Through the practice of aromatherapy, we can live better lives and become better people!

Thank you again for downloading this book! I hope it was able to provide you genuine value!

Finally, if you enjoyed this book and believe that it can serve and provide value to others, please leave feedback to help promote and support our goal of helping more and more readers! Afterwards please take a moment to check out my other books as well as join my Free Newsletter for Free Bonus Content! (Details on following pages.)

Flip past the final page of this book to leave a review on Amazon!

Thank you and good luck!

Check Out My Other Books & Join My Free Newsletter!

Below you'll find some of my other popular books that are popular on Amazon and Kindle as well. Simply click on the links below to check them out. Alternatively, you can visit my author page on Amazon: www.amazon.com/author/cassandraslain

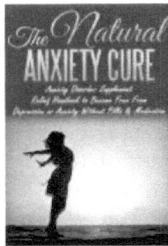 **Natural Anxiety Cure:** http://amzn.to/1Jx86Zl

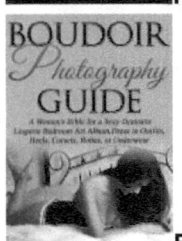 **Boudoir Photography Guide:** http://amzn.to/1AUynOl

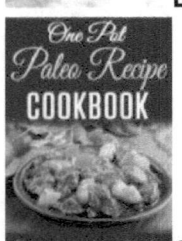 **One Pot Paleo Recipe Cookbook:** http://amzn.to/1dWBgo1

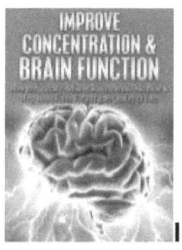**Improve Concentration & Brain Function:**
http://amzn.to/1QCyMXM

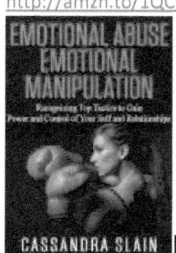Emotional Abuse & Emotional Manipulation:
http://amzn.to/1Kn5woj

Join My Free Newsletter!: http://eepurl.com/bpHpdH

www.ingramcontent.com/pod-product-compliance
Lightning Source LLC
Chambersburg PA
CBHW021001180526
45163CB00006B/2450